Journey to the

A Comprehensive Travel Guide to Machu Picchu

Carlos Dylan

Table of Contents

Chapter One
Introduction
- About Machu Picchu   6
- Brief History and Significance   9
- Why Visit Machu Picchu?   13

Chapter Two
Planning Your Trip
- Best Time to Visit   18
- Entry Requirements and Permits   20
- Choosing the Right Tour or Trek   23
- Packing Essentials   27

Chapter Three
Getting There
- Arriving in Peru   32
- Transportation Options to Machu Picchu   35
- Cusco: Gateway to Machu Picchu   38
- Train Rides to Aguas Calientes   41

Chapter Four
Exploring Aguas Calientes
- Overview of the Town   46
- Accommodation Options   49
- Dining and Local Cuisine   52

- Shopping and Souvenirs   55

Chapter Five
Machu Picchu Treks and Routes
- Inca Trail: Classic Route   60
- Salkantay Trek: Alternative Route 63
- Other Trekking Options   66

Chapter Six
Guided Tours and Independent Exploration
- Pros and Cons of Guided Tours   70
- Tips for Exploring Independently 73
- Hiring Local Guides   77

Chapter Seven
The Magnificence of Machu Picchu
- Arriving at Machu Picchu   82
- Layout and Key Structures   85
- Sun Gate and Inti Punku   88

Chapter Eight
Cultural and Natural Highlights
- Temples and Religious Sites   92
- Agricultural Terraces   95
- Natural Surroundings and Scenic Views   98

Chapter Nine
Photography Tips
- Best Photo Spots   102
- Capturing Sunrise and Sunset   105
- Recommended Gear   108

Chapter Ten
Respecting the Site
- Sustainable Tourism Practices   112
- Leave No Trace Principles   115
- Cultural Sensitivity   117

Chapter Eleven
Additional Attractions Nearby
- Huayna Picchu Hike   122
- Machu Picchu Mountain Hike   124
- Hot Springs at Aguas Calientes   127

Chapter Twelve
Practical Information
- Safety and Health Considerations 132
- Language and Communication   135
- Currency and Banking   138
- Useful Phrases   141

Chapter Thirteen
Resources and Contacts

- Travel Agencies and Tour Operators 146
- Official Websites and Resources 149
- Emergency Contacts 152

Appendix
- Recommended Reading and Films 156

CHAPTER ONE
INTRODUCTION

1.1 About Machu Picchu

Machu Picchu is an ancient Incan citadel located high in the Andes Mountains of Peru. It is one of the most iconic and well-preserved archaeological sites in the world, often referred to as the "Lost City of the Incas." The site's stunning beauty, architectural marvels, and mysterious history have made it a UNESCO World Heritage Site and one of the New Seven Wonders of the World.

Key Features and Characteristics:

Architectural Marvels: Machu Picchu showcases the incredible engineering skills of the Inca civilization. The site features finely crafted stone structures, terraced fields, ceremonial plazas, temples, and intricate stone pathways.

Terracing and Agriculture: The Incas ingeniously adapted the steep mountain terrain to create terraced fields for agricultural purposes. These terraces were used for cultivating crops like maize, quinoa, and potatoes.

Inti Watana: A ritual stone known as the "Hitching Post of the Sun," believed to have been used for astronomical and ritualistic purposes.

Temple of the Sun: A semi-circular tower with precisely carved stone blocks, possibly used for astronomical observations and rituals related to the sun.

Royal Residence: The complex contains living quarters, possibly used by the Inca ruler or elite individuals, adorned with intricate stonework.

Sacred Rock: A massive stone with symbolic carvings, believed to have held spiritual significance.

Stunning Views: Machu Picchu offers breathtaking panoramic views of the surrounding mountains and the Urubamba River valley.

Historical Significance:

The exact purpose of Machu Picchu remains a subject of scholarly debate. It is thought to have been built in the mid-15th century during the height of the Inca Empire under the rule of Emperor Pachacuti. Some theories suggest it was a royal estate, a religious center, or a retreat for Inca nobility.

Discovery and Preservation:

Machu Picchu remained relatively unknown to the outside world until its rediscovery by American historian and explorer Hiram Bingham in 1911. Since then, it has captivated travelers, historians, and archaeologists alike. Efforts have been made to preserve and protect the site from the effects of tourism and environmental factors.

Visiting Machu Picchu:

To visit Machu Picchu, travelers typically start their journey from the nearby town of Aguas Calientes. Options for reaching the site include hiking the famous Inca Trail or taking a train. Entry to Machu Picchu requires a valid ticket and, in some cases, permits for specific treks.

Cultural and Spiritual Significance:

Machu Picchu continues to hold cultural and spiritual significance for modern-day Peruvians, as well as global visitors. Its unique blend of historical importance, architectural marvels, and natural beauty makes it a must-visit destination for anyone interested in history, archaeology, and breathtaking landscapes

1.2 Brief History and Significance

Machu Picchu, often referred to as the "Lost City of the Incas," is an ancient citadel situated atop the Andes Mountains in Peru.

Its history and significance are intertwined with the rise and fall of the Inca Empire: Inca Civilization (15th Century): Machu Picchu is believed to have been built during the mid-15th century, around the time of Emperor Pachacuti, a powerful Inca ruler. The exact purpose of the site is still debated among historians, but it is thought to have served as a royal estate, a ceremonial center, or a religious sanctuary.

Abandonment and Rediscovery: As the Inca Empire faced upheavals and external pressures, including the Spanish conquest, Machu Picchu was eventually abandoned, likely in the late 16th century. The site remained hidden from the outside world for centuries, concealed by the dense vegetation of the Andean cloud forest.

Rediscovery (1911): In 1911, American historian and explorer Hiram Bingham, with the assistance of local guides, stumbled upon Machu Picchu. His efforts to document and excavate the site brought it to international attention. Bingham's work contributed significantly to understanding Inca history and culture.

Archaeological Significance: Machu Picchu's architectural brilliance is a testament to the advanced engineering and construction skills of the Inca civilization. The precise fitting of massive stone blocks without the use of mortar, the sophisticated terracing for agriculture, and the alignment of structures with celestial events showcase the Incas' deep understanding of architecture, astronomy, and culture.

UNESCO World Heritage Site (1983): In recognition of its cultural and historical importance, Machu Picchu was designated a UNESCO World Heritage Site in 1983. The designation emphasizes the need for its preservation and protection.

Tourism and Conservation Challenges: Machu Picchu's popularity as a global tourist destination has presented both opportunities and challenges. While tourism brings economic benefits to the local communities and the country, it also places strain on the site's delicate ecosystem and historic structures. Conservation efforts aim to strike a balance between facilitating tourism and safeguarding the site's integrity.

Cultural and Symbolic Value: Machu Picchu holds immense cultural and symbolic value for modern-day Peruvians, who view it as a link to their ancestral heritage and a symbol of national pride. It represents the resilience and ingenuity of the Inca civilization in the face of historical changes.

Preserving the Legacy: Efforts are ongoing to protect and preserve Machu Picchu for future generations. Measures include limiting the number of daily visitors, implementing sustainable tourism practices, and conducting ongoing research to better understand the site's history and significance.

1.3 Why Visit Machu Picchu

Visiting Machu Picchu offers a unique and unforgettable experience that combines historical, cultural, and natural wonders. Here are some compelling reasons to visit Machu Picchu:

1. Architectural Marvel: Witness the astonishing architectural achievements of the Inca civilization. The precision-cut stone blocks, intricate terracing, and complex layout showcase the advanced engineering skills of the time.

2. Historical Significance: Explore the mysteries and history of the Inca Empire. Machu Picchu provides a glimpse into the daily life, rituals, and beliefs of this ancient civilization.

3. Breathtaking Views: Enjoy awe-inspiring panoramic views of the Andes Mountains and the Urubamba River valley. The stunning natural beauty surrounding Machu Picchu adds to the site's allure.

4. Cultural Immersion: Immerse yourself in the rich cultural heritage of Peru. Learn about the Inca traditions, customs, and architectural techniques that have left an indelible mark on the region.

5. Spiritual Connection: Experience the spiritual atmosphere that permeates Machu Picchu. Many visitors describe a sense of reverence and connection to the past while exploring the site.

6. Bucket-List Destination: Machu Picchu is often regarded as one of the must-visit destinations in the world, making it an essential addition to any traveler's bucket list.

7. Hiking and Adventure: Embark on legendary treks like the Inca Trail or the Salkantay Trek to reach Machu Picchu. These journeys offer not only a physical challenge but also a deeper connection to the land.

8. Photography Opportunities: Capture stunning photographs of the iconic site, its

architectural details, and the surrounding landscapes during sunrise and sunset.

9. Educational Experience: Gain insights into Inca history, architecture, and culture through guided tours and interpretive displays at the site.

10. Personal Achievement: Standing amidst the ancient ruins and taking in the breathtaking scenery can evoke a sense of accomplishment and wonder, creating lasting memories.

11. Supporting Local Communities: Tourism contributes to the local economy, benefiting nearby communities and helping preserve the cultural heritage of the region.

12. Adventure and Discovery: Whether you arrive by train or on foot, the journey to Machu Picchu is an adventure in itself, filled with discoveries and memorable experiences.

13. UNESCO World Heritage Site: Experience the honor of visiting a UNESCO

World Heritage Site that is recognized globally for its cultural and historical significance.

14. Connection with Nature: The journey to Machu Picchu often involves traversing diverse landscapes, from dense forests to high mountain passes, providing a unique opportunity to connect with nature.

CHAPTER TWO
PLANNING YOUR TRIP

2.1 Best time to visit

The best times to visit Machu Picchu depend on various factors, including weather, crowds, and personal preferences. Here are the two main seasons to consider:

1. Dry Season (May to September): This is generally considered the best time to visit Machu Picchu due to the dry weather and clearer skies. May to August are the peak months with the lowest chances of rain, making it ideal for trekking and exploring. The weather is cooler, especially at higher altitudes, so be prepared for chilly nights. However, because of the favorable conditions, this is also the busiest time at Machu Picchu. It's advisable to book your accommodations and permits well in advance.

2. Wet Season (October to April): The wet season corresponds to the summer months

in the Southern Hemisphere. While there is a higher chance of rain and cloud cover, the landscape is lush and green, creating beautiful photo opportunities. Fewer tourists visit during this time, which means you might have a more tranquil experience at the site. The Inca Trail is closed for maintenance during February, and some treks might be affected by heavy rainfall and landslides. If you're willing to accept some rain and are interested in a less crowded experience, visiting during the wet season can be rewarding.

Considerations:

1. Peak Crowds: June to August is the busiest period due to the combination of dry weather and summer vacations. If you prefer a quieter experience, you might want to visit in the shoulder seasons of May or September.

2. Weather: The dry season offers more predictable weather, but the wet season has its own charm with lush landscapes. Be

prepared for rain if you visit during the wet season.

3. Availability: If you plan to hike the Inca Trail, be aware that permits can sell out quickly, especially during the peak season. Booking well in advance is crucial.

4. Altitude: Machu Picchu is located at a high altitude, and weather conditions can vary significantly. Pack clothing that can accommodate both warm and cool temperatures.

5. Personal Preferences: Consider whether you prioritize clear views and dry conditions or a more serene and less crowded atmosphere.

2.2 Entry Requirements and Permits

Entry requirements and permits for visiting Machu Picchu can vary depending on your travel plans, whether you're visiting the citadel only or also planning to hike one of the surrounding trails. Here's a general overview of entry requirements and permits:

1. Machu Picchu Entrance Ticket: All visitors to Machu Picchu, regardless of whether they are hiking or not, need to purchase an entrance ticket. Tickets can be purchased online in advance through the official government website or at authorized ticket offices in Cusco or Aguas Calientes (Machu Picchu Pueblo). It is recommended to buy your entrance ticket in advance, especially during the high tourist season, to secure your desired entry date and time.

2. Hiking Permits (Inca Trail and Other Treks): If you plan to hike the classic Inca Trail or other alternative treks like the Salkantay Trek, Lares Trek, or Choquequirao Trek, you'll need specific hiking permits. These permits have limited availability and should be secured well in advance, sometimes several months ahead, especially for the Inca Trail. The hiking permits typically include the entrance to Machu Picchu as part of the trek.

3. Huayna Picchu and Machu Picchu Mountain: If you wish to hike Huayna Picchu or Machu Picchu Mountain, both of which offer panoramic views of the site, you'll need additional permits. These permits are separate from the entrance ticket and often have limited availability. It's recommended to book them in advance.

4. Passport Information: When purchasing tickets, you'll likely need to provide your passport information. Make sure your passport is valid for at least six months from the date of entry. There might also be additional health and safety protocols in place.

5. Tour Operators and Agencies: If you're joining a guided tour or working with a travel agency, they can often assist you in obtaining the necessary permits and tickets.

2.3 Choosing the Right Tour or Trek

Choosing the right tour or trek to Machu Picchu is an important decision that depends on your interests, fitness level, time constraints, and preferred level of adventure. Below are some factors to consider when making your choice:

1. Type of Trek
Classic Inca Trail: This is the most famous and iconic trek to Machu Picchu, known for its historical significance and stunning scenery. It typically requires booking well in advance due to limited permits.
Alternative Treks: There are several alternative treks, such as the Salkantay Trek, Lares Trek, and Choquequirao Trek, each offering unique experiences and landscapes. These treks are often less crowded than the Inca Trail.

2. Duration: The length of the trek can vary significantly. The Inca Trail is usually around 4 days, while some alternative treks can be shorter or longer. Consider how

much time you have available for your journey.

3. Fitness Level: Some treks, like the Inca Trail, involve challenging uphill and downhill sections, high altitudes, and long distances. Make sure you choose a trek that matches your fitness level and hiking experience.

4. Altitude Acclimatization: If you're not accustomed to high altitudes, it's a good idea to choose a trek that allows for proper acclimatization to minimize the risk of altitude sickness.

5. Scenery and Terrain: Research the landscapes and terrain of each trek to find one that aligns with your preferences. Some treks pass through diverse ecosystems, including mountains, jungles, and traditional villages.

6. Camping vs. Lodges: Consider whether you prefer camping or staying in lodges along the route. The Inca Trail involves

camping, while some alternative treks offer lodge-to-lodge options.

7. Group vs. Solo Trek: Decide whether you want to join a group trek or go solo. Group treks can provide camaraderie and support, while solo treks offer more flexibility and solitude.

8. Tour Operator and Guides: Choose a reputable tour operator with experienced guides who can enhance your trekking experience with insights into the history, culture, and nature of the region.

9. Permit Availability: If you have a specific trek in mind, check the availability of permits. The Inca Trail, for example, has limited permits and requires booking well in advance.

10. Budget: Different treks have varying costs, which may include entrance fees, permits, transportation, guides, meals, and accommodations. Consider your budget when making your decision.

11. Season and Weather: Consider the time of year you're planning to visit. The dry season (May to September) offers clearer weather, while the wet season (October to April) is less crowded.

12. Personal Preferences: Ultimately, choose a trek that aligns with your personal preferences, whether you're seeking historical insights, natural beauty, physical challenges, or a combination of these factors.

Research thoroughly, read reviews, and consult with experienced trekkers or travel experts to make an informed decision. Remember that whichever trek you choose, the journey to Machu Picchu is a once-in-a-lifetime experience that will leave you with incredible memories and a deeper appreciation for the region's rich history and culture.

2.4 Packing Essentials

When preparing for a trek or visit to Machu Picchu, it's crucial to pack thoughtfully to ensure your comfort, safety, and enjoyment. Below is a list of packing essentials to consider:

1. Moisture-Wicking Clothing: Choose lightweight, moisture-wicking clothing to stay dry and comfortable during hikes.

2. Layering System: Pack clothing in layers to adjust to varying temperatures. Include a mix of short-sleeve and long-sleeve shirts, a fleece or sweater, and a waterproof jacket.

3. Hiking Pants and Shorts: Opt for comfortable, quick-drying hiking pants and shorts.

4. Undergarments and Socks: Bring moisture-wicking underwear and several pairs of hiking socks.

5. Warm Hat and Gloves: Essential for colder mornings or high altitudes.

6. Hiking Boots: Sturdy, waterproof hiking boots with good ankle support are essential for trekking.

7. Comfortable Shoes: Lightweight and comfortable shoes for wearing around camp or during leisure time.

8. Backpack: A comfortable, well-fitting backpack to carry your essentials during the trek.

9. Sleeping Bag: Choose a sleeping bag suitable for the expected temperatures during your trek.

10. Sleeping Pad: An inflatable or foam sleeping pad for added comfort.

11. Trekking Poles: Helpful for balance and reducing strain on your knees, especially during descents.

12. Headlamp or Flashlight: Useful for early morning starts and navigating in the dark.

13. Sun Protection: Sunscreen, sunglasses with UV protection, and a wide-brimmed hat to shield yourself from the sun.

14. Insect Repellent: Protect yourself from mosquitoes and other insects, especially in humid areas.

15. Toiletries: Include travel-sized toiletries such as toothbrush, toothpaste, biodegradable soap, and a small towel.

16. Personal Medications: Carry any necessary prescription medications, along with a basic first aid kit.

17. Reusable Water Bottle: Stay hydrated by carrying a refillable water bottle and consider water purification tablets or a water filter.

18. Snacks: Energy bars, trail mix, and other lightweight snacks for sustenance during hikes.

19. Camera and Binoculars: Capture the stunning scenery and wildlife, and binoculars for bird watching.

20. Travel Documents: Passport, tickets, permits, and any necessary travel insurance information.

21. Cash: Bring local currency for small purchases and tips.

22. Walking Stick or Trekking Poles: Especially helpful for individuals with knee or joint concerns.

23. Camera Equipment: If you're a photography enthusiast, pack your camera gear.

24. Portable Charger: Keep your devices charged, especially if you plan to use your smartphone for navigation or photography.

CHAPTER THREE
GETTING THERE

3.1 Arriving in Peru

Arriving in Peru for a visit to Machu Picchu involves several steps, including international travel, arrival in Lima (the capital city), and subsequent travel to Cusco or Aguas Calientes (Machu Picchu Pueblo). Here's a general overview of what to expect upon arriving in Peru:

1. International Flight:
- Book a flight to Jorge Chávez International Airport (LIM) in Lima, Peru. This is the main international airport in the country.
- Complete any required customs and immigration procedures upon arrival.

2. Arrival in Lima:
- Upon disembarking, follow signs to immigration, where you will present your passport, completed immigration form, and any required visa (if applicable).

- Collect your luggage at the baggage claim area.

3. Transit in Lima (Optional):
- Depending on your travel plans, you may have a layover in Lima before your onward flight to Cusco or other destinations. Some travelers choose to explore Lima for a day or two before continuing their journey.

4. Domestic Flight to Cusco:
- If you're heading directly to Cusco, you'll need to book a domestic flight from Lima to Alejandro Velasco Astete International Airport (CUZ) in Cusco. This is the main airport closest to Machu Picchu.
- Allow for some time between your international and domestic flights to account for any potential delays.

5. Arrival in Cusco:
- After landing in Cusco, follow signs to immigration and collect your luggage.
- The city of Cusco is located at high altitude, so it's important to take it easy upon arrival to acclimate to the altitude.

6. Transport to Aguas Calientes (Machu Picchu Pueblo):
- From Cusco, you'll need to travel to Aguas Calientes, the gateway town to Machu Picchu. The most common way to reach Aguas Calientes is by taking a train from Cusco or Ollantaytambo.
- Alternatively, you can embark on a multi-day trek to Machu Picchu, such as the Inca Trail or an alternative trek.

7. Accommodation:
- Once you arrive in Aguas Calientes, check into your chosen accommodation. Make sure you have your reservation details handy.

8. Next-Day Machu Picchu Visit:
- If you plan to visit Machu Picchu the following day, make sure you have your entrance ticket and any required permits ready. You'll need to arrange transportation to the entrance of Machu Picchu from Aguas Calientes, either by bus or on foot.

9. Enjoy Your Visit to Machu Picchu: Take in the breathtaking sights and explore the ancient ruins of Machu Picchu.

3.2 Transportation Options to Machu Picchu

There are several transportation options to reach Machu Picchu, each offering a different experience and level of convenience. Here are the main transportation options available:

1. Train: The train is one of the most popular and convenient ways to get to Machu Picchu. Trains operate from the town of Ollantaytambo or Poroy (near Cusco) to Aguas Calientes, the nearest town to Machu Picchu. Different train services offer various levels of comfort and amenities, ranging from economy class to luxury options. The train journey provides stunning views of the Andean landscapes along the way.

2. Hiking/Trekking: Hiking to Machu Picchu is a rewarding and adventurous option. The most famous trek is the Inca Trail, which requires permits and must be booked in advance. It typically takes about 4 days to complete. There are alternative treks, such as the Salkantay Trek, Lares Trek, and Choquequirao Trek, each offering unique landscapes and experiences.

3. Bus and Walk: From Aguas Calientes, you can take a shuttle bus to the entrance of Machu Picchu. After the bus drop-off point, there is a short uphill walk to the entrance gate. The walk takes about 15-20 minutes and includes a steep set of stairs.

4. Helicopter: For a truly unique and scenic experience, you can opt for a helicopter tour to Machu Picchu. Helicopter tours typically depart from Cusco or the Sacred Valley.

5. Biking: Some tour operators offer biking tours that combine biking with other modes of transportation, such as trains or buses, to reach Machu Picchu.

6. Combination Tours: Many tour operators offer combination packages that include a mix of transportation modes, such as train and bus, for a comprehensive and varied experience.

Important Tips:

Advance Planning: Depending on your chosen transportation option, you might need to book tickets or permits well in advance, especially during peak seasons.

Altitude Considerations: Machu Picchu is located at a relatively high altitude. Take time to acclimate to the altitude before embarking on any treks or activities.

Weather Preparedness: Be prepared for various weather conditions, including rain, sun, and cold temperatures, especially in the early mornings and evenings.

Local Regulations: Respect local regulations, follow guidelines, and practice responsible tourism to help preserve this iconic site.

3.3 Cusco: Gateway to Machu Picchu

Cusco, often referred to as the "Gateway to Machu Picchu," is a vibrant and historically rich city located in the Andes Mountains of Peru. It serves as a popular starting point for travelers on their journey to the iconic Inca citadel. Here's a closer look at Cusco and its significance as the gateway to Machu Picchu:

1. Inca Capital: Cusco was the capital of the Inca Empire and held immense importance as the center of political, religious, and administrative activities. Many of its streets and buildings still bear the marks of Inca craftsmanship.

2. Colonial Influence: After the Spanish conquest, Cusco underwent significant transformation. Spanish colonial architecture blended with Inca foundations, creating a unique urban landscape.

3. Cultural Heritage: The city is a UNESCO World Heritage Site, recognized for its historical and architectural significance. It's

a living testament to the blend of Inca and Spanish cultures.

Attractions and Highlights:

1. Plaza de Armas: Cusco's main square is a bustling hub surrounded by historic buildings, churches, and restaurants. It's an excellent starting point for exploring the city.

2. Cathedral of Santo Domingo: This grand cathedral was built on the foundations of the Inca temple of Koricancha, showcasing the juxtaposition of Inca and Spanish influences.

3. Sacsayhuaman: A remarkable Inca archaeological site located on the outskirts of Cusco. Its massive stone walls and panoramic views of the city are awe-inspiring.

4. Qorikancha: The Inca Temple of the Sun, a stunning example of Inca stonework, is located within the Santo Domingo Convent.

5. San Pedro Market: Immerse yourself in local life by visiting this bustling market where you can find fresh produce, traditional crafts, and a variety of local goods.

6. Chinchero: A charming village near Cusco known for its traditional weaving techniques and Inca ruins.

Gateway to Machu Picchu:

1. Starting Point: Many travelers begin their journey to Machu Picchu from Cusco. The city's well-developed infrastructure and transportation connections make it a convenient base.

2. Acclimatization: Cusco's altitude (3,400 meters or 11,150 feet) offers an opportunity for visitors to acclimate to the high altitude before embarking on treks or visiting Machu Picchu.

3. Train Departures: Cusco is a departure point for trains that take visitors to Aguas Calientes, the town located near Machu

Picchu. From Aguas Calientes, travelers can take a bus or hike to the citadel.

4. Inca Trail: For those embarking on the Inca Trail trek to Machu Picchu, Cusco is the initial starting point and serves as a hub for tour operators and preparations.

3.4 Train Rides to Aguas Calientes

Taking a train ride to Aguas Calientes is one of the most popular and convenient ways to reach the gateway to Machu Picchu. Here's a guide to the train rides to Aguas Calientes, which is the town closest to Machu Picchu:

Train Stations:
1. Poroy Station (Cusco): Located about 20-30 minutes from Cusco by taxi or shuttle, this station offers train services to Aguas Calientes.

2. Ollantaytambo Station: This station is located in the town of Ollantaytambo, which is about a 2-hour drive from Cusco.

Many travelers choose to start their train journey from here.

Train Services:

Several train companies operate services between Cusco (or Ollantaytambo) and Aguas Calientes. Each offers varying levels of comfort and amenities. Some of the prominent train services include:

1. PeruRail: PeruRail offers different train classes, including Expedition, Vistadome, and the luxurious Belmond Hiram Bingham train.
   - Expedition: A comfortable option with panoramic windows and light refreshments.
   - Vistadome: Upgraded service with larger windows, entertainment, and snacks.
   - Belmond Hiram Bingham: An elegant and luxurious experience with fine dining, live music, and guided tours.

2. Inca Rail:

- Inca Rail also offers different classes, such as the Voyager and the 360° Train.
- Voyager: Comfortable seats, panoramic windows, and light snacks.
- 360° Train: Features large windows and glass ceilings for optimal views.

Ticket Booking and Reservations: It is advisable to book your train tickets in advance, especially during peak seasons, as they can sell out quickly. Tickets can be purchased directly from the train company's website or through authorized agents.

Scenic Views: The train journey from Cusco (or Ollantaytambo) to Aguas Calientes offers breathtaking views of the Andean landscapes, including lush valleys, towering mountains, and rushing rivers. Many of the train cars have large windows, providing excellent opportunities for photography and enjoying the scenery.

Duration and Schedule: The train ride from Poroy or Ollantaytambo to Aguas Calientes takes approximately 3 to 4 hours, depending on the service and route. Train schedules may vary based on the company and the time of year. Trains typically depart in the morning and early afternoon.

Aguas Calientes: Upon arriving in Aguas Calientes, you can explore the town, relax in hot springs (which gave the town its name), and prepare for your visit to Machu Picchu the following day. Taking a train ride to Aguas Calientes is a comfortable and scenic way to begin your Machu Picchu adventure. It allows you to enjoy the journey while taking in the beauty of the Peruvian landscapes.

CHAPTER FOUR
EXPLORING AGUAS CALIENTES

4.1 Overview of the Town

Aguas Calientes, also known as Machu Picchu Pueblo, is a small town nestled in the Andes Mountains of Peru. It serves as the gateway to the iconic Machu Picchu archaeological site. Here's an overview of Aguas Calientes and what you can expect when visiting:

Location and Accessibility: Aguas Calientes is located at the base of the mountains that lead up to Machu Picchu, making it the closest town to the archaeological site. The town is not accessible by road; visitors typically arrive by train from Cusco or Ollantaytambo and then take a short bus ride or hike to Machu Picchu.

Characteristics: Aguas Calientes is a small and bustling town with a distinct atmosphere. It has a mix of local culture and international influence due to its status as a popular tourist destination. The town is surrounded by lush vegetation, and the Urubamba River flows through it.

Attractions and Activities:

1. Hot Springs: The town is named after its natural hot springs, which are a popular attraction. Visitors can relax and unwind in these thermal baths after a day of exploring Machu Picchu or hiking.

2. Craft Markets: Aguas Calientes has a range of artisan markets and souvenir shops where you can find traditional Peruvian crafts, textiles, jewelry, and more.

3. Restaurants and Dining: The town offers a variety of dining options, ranging from local Peruvian cuisine to international fare. It's a good place to try traditional dishes or refuel after a day of exploration.

4. Gateway to Machu Picchu: Aguas Calientes is the starting point for most visitors to Machu Picchu. From here, you can take a shuttle bus or hike up to the entrance of the archaeological site.

Accommodation: Aguas Calientes has a range of accommodations, including hotels, hostels, and lodges catering to various budgets. It's a good idea to book your accommodation in advance, especially during peak tourist seasons.

Practical Tips:
1. Weather: The weather in Aguas Calientes can be unpredictable. Pack clothing for both warm and cool conditions, and be prepared for rain.

2. Altitude: While Aguas Calientes is at a lower altitude than Cusco, it's still advisable to take it easy and acclimate to the altitude before exploring Machu Picchu.

3. Early Start: Many visitors stay in Aguas Calientes the night before their visit to Machu Picchu to ensure an early start. The first buses to Machu Picchu depart in the early morning.

4. Limited Services: Keep in mind that due to its remote location, services in Aguas

Calientes might not be as extensive as in larger cities.

4.2 Accomodation Options

Aguas Calientes, the gateway to Machu Picchu, offers a variety of accommodation options to suit different budgets and preferences. Here are some types of lodging you can consider when staying in Aguas Calientes:

1. Hotels and Resorts: Aguas Calientes has a range of hotels and resorts, ranging from budget to luxury. These establishments offer various amenities, including comfortable rooms, restaurants, and sometimes spa facilities. Luxury hotels may offer stunning views of the surrounding mountains and the Urubamba River.

2. Hostels and Guesthouses: For budget-conscious travelers, hostels and guesthouses provide affordable accommodation options. These places

typically offer dormitory-style rooms or private rooms with shared facilities. Hostels are often popular among backpackers and solo travelers looking for a social atmosphere.

3. Boutique Lodges: Some lodges in Aguas Calientes offer a boutique experience with personalized service, unique decor, and a cozy ambiance.

4. Eco-Lodges: If you're interested in a more eco-friendly experience, some lodges focus on sustainability and environmental conservation.

5. Lodges with Thermal Baths: Some lodges have their own thermal baths, allowing guests to enjoy hot springs without leaving the property.

6. Online Booking Platforms: Websites and platforms like Booking.com, Expedia, TripAdvisor, and Airbnb can help you find and compare various accommodation options in Aguas Calientes.

Tips for Choosing Accommodation:

1. Location: Consider how close the accommodation is to the train station and bus stop, as well as its proximity to Machu Picchu. Some lodgings offer easy access, while others might require a short walk or transportation.

2. Amenities: Check for amenities that are important to you, such as Wi-Fi, hot water, breakfast, and on-site restaurants.

3. Reviews: Read reviews from previous guests to get an idea of the quality of service, cleanliness, and overall experience at the accommodation.

4. Price: Aguas Calientes offers options for various budgets. Determine how much you're willing to spend and look for accommodations within that range.

5. Reservations: Especially during peak tourist seasons, it's a good idea to make reservations in advance to secure your preferred lodging.

6. Group Size: If you're traveling with a group, consider accommodations that can accommodate multiple people comfortably.

4.3 Dining and Local Cuisine

Dining in Aguas Calientes offers a variety of options to satisfy different tastes and preferences. You'll find a mix of local Peruvian cuisine, international dishes, and traditional Andean flavors. Here's an overview of dining and local cuisine in Aguas Calientes:

Local Cuisine:
Peruvian cuisine is known for its diverse and flavorful dishes, often showcasing a blend of indigenous ingredients and influences from Spanish, African, Asian, and other cuisines. In Aguas Calientes, you can try some of the following local dishes:

1. Ceviche:Fresh seafood (often fish or shrimp) marinated in lime juice and served with onions, peppers, and cilantro.

2. Lomo Saltado: A stir-fry dish made with marinated beef, onions, tomatoes, and fries, often served with rice.

3. Aji de Gallina: Shredded chicken cooked in a creamy sauce made with aji amarillo peppers, cheese, and nuts.

4. Pachamanca: A traditional Andean dish featuring marinated meats and vegetables cooked in an underground oven.

5. Quinoa Soup: A nutritious soup made with quinoa, vegetables, and sometimes cheese or meat.

6. Alpaca Steak: A unique protein option, alpaca meat is lean and tender, often served grilled or in a sauce.

7. Andean Potatoes: Try various types of native potatoes prepared in different ways, such as boiled, fried, or mashed.

Dining Options in Aguas Calientes:

1. Local Restaurants: Many local restaurants in Aguas Calientes offer traditional Peruvian dishes, as well as international options.

2. Pizzerias and Cafés: You'll find a number of pizzerias and cafés offering pizzas, sandwiches, and coffee.

3. Street Food: Look for street vendors selling snacks like empanadas, tamales, and sweet treats.

4. Market Eateries: The local market might have food stalls where you can enjoy affordable and authentic Peruvian meals.

5. Upscale Dining: Some hotels and lodges offer upscale dining experiences, often with a focus on fresh, locally sourced ingredients.

Tips for Dining:
1. Local Specialties: Don't hesitate to ask the staff for recommendations on local dishes or specialties.

2. Vegetarian and Vegan Options: Many restaurants offer vegetarian and vegan choices to accommodate different dietary preferences.

3. Bottled Water: It is advisable to drink bottled water to stay hydrated, especially if you're not accustomed to the local water.

4. Reservations: During peak tourist seasons, popular restaurants might get busy. Consider making reservations in advance.

5. Culinary Tours: Some guided culinary tours in Aguas Calientes allow you to explore local markets, learn about traditional cooking techniques, and enjoy a hands-on cooking experience.

4.4 Shopping and Souvenirs

Aguas Calientes offers a range of shopping opportunities, allowing you to bring home unique souvenirs and mementos that reflect the local culture and heritage. Here's a guide to shopping and finding souvenirs in Aguas Calientes:

1. Souvenir Shops: The town has numerous souvenir shops where you can find a variety of items, including textiles, clothing, ceramics, jewelry, and more.Look for handmade crafts, such as alpaca wool clothing, scarves, hats, and gloves. These items showcase traditional Peruvian weaving techniques and designs.

2. Alpaca Products: Alpaca wool is a popular material used to make clothing, accessories, and textiles. Look for soft and luxurious alpaca sweaters, blankets, and scarves.

3. Andean Crafts: Traditional Andean crafts like intricately woven textiles, colorful ponchos, hand-carved wooden items, and pottery can be great additions to your collection.

4. Silver Jewelry: Peru is known for its high-quality silver craftsmanship. You can

find unique silver jewelry pieces featuring indigenous designs and motifs.

5. Musical Instruments: Look for small musical instruments like panpipes (zampoñas) and charangos, which are traditional Andean instruments often used in local music.

6. Local Artwork: Some shops offer paintings, prints, and other forms of local artwork that capture the beauty of the region.

7. Andean Musical Instruments:bLook for small musical instruments like panpipes (zampoñas) and charangos, which are traditional Andean instruments often used in local music.

8. Coffee and Chocolate: Aguas Calientes is also known for its coffee and chocolate. You can find local coffee beans and chocolate products that make for great gifts.

Tips for Shopping:

1. Bargaining: Bargaining is not as common in formal stores, but you can try it at local markets and stalls. Always do so with respect and a friendly attitude.

2. Quality: When purchasing textiles or crafts, examine the quality of the materials and workmanship to ensure you're getting an authentic and well-made product.

3. Support Local Artisans: Many shops support local artisans and offer handmade products. By purchasing from these establishments, you contribute to the local economy and support traditional crafts.

4. Authenticity: Look for shops that showcase the work of local artists and artisans to ensure that you're purchasing authentic and locally crafted items.

5. Cultural Sensitivity: When shopping for clothing or items with indigenous designs, be mindful of cultural sensitivity and the significance of these designs to the local communities.

CHAPTER FIVE
MACHU PICCHU TREKS AND ROUTES

5.1 Inca Trail: Classic Route

The Inca Trail is one of the most famous and iconic trekking routes in the world, leading to the ancient citadel of Machu Picchu. The classic Inca Trail route is a 4-day, 3-night trek that offers breathtaking landscapes, archaeological sites, and a sense of adventure. Here's an overview of the classic Inca Trail route:

Day 1: Cusco - Piskacucho (KM 82) - Wayllabamba:
- Start the trek at the trailhead near Piskacucho (KM 82), following the Urubamba River.
- Pass through small villages, enjoy scenic views, and witness the archaeological site of Llactapata.
- Camp overnight at the village of Wayllabamba.

Day 2: Wayllabamba - Dead Woman's Pass
- Pacaymayo:
- Begin the steep ascent to Dead Woman's
Pass (Warmiwañusca) at an altitude of
about 4,215 meters (13,828 feet).
- Descend to the Pacaymayo Valley and
camp near Pacaymayo.

Day 3: Pacaymayo - Phuyupatamarca -
Wiñay Wayna:
- Pass through the second pass,
Runkurakay (3,950 meters/12,959 feet),
and visit the archaeological site of
Sayacmarca.
- Trek through cloud forests, enjoy
stunning views, and reach the third pass,
Phuyupatamarca (3,680 meters/12,073
feet).
- Descend to Wiñay Wayna, an impressive
Inca site, and camp nearby.

Day 4: Wiñay Wayna - Machu Picchu -
Aguas Calientes:
- Begin early to reach the Sun Gate (Inti
Punku) and witness the sunrise over Machu
Picchu.

- Descend to Machu Picchu for a guided tour of the archaeological site.
- In the afternoon, take a bus or hike down to Aguas Calientes, where you can relax and unwind.

Additional Information:
- The classic Inca Trail requires a permit, and these permits often sell out quickly, so it's essential to book well in advance through a licensed tour operator.
- The trek involves hiking at high altitudes, so acclimatization is crucial. Spending a few days in Cusco before the trek is recommended.
- The trail offers stunning views of the Andean landscapes, diverse ecosystems, and impressive Inca ruins along the way.
- Trekkers camp in designated campsites with basic facilities. Porters often carry much of the camping and cooking equipment.
- The classic Inca Trail offers a challenging and rewarding experience, allowing you to connect with the ancient past and culminating in the awe-inspiring arrival at Machu Picchu.

5.2 Salkantay Trek: Alternative Route

The Salkantay Trek is a popular alternative route to Machu Picchu, offering a diverse and challenging trekking experience through stunning landscapes. This trek is known for its impressive views of the Salkantay Mountain, diverse ecosystems, and opportunities to connect with local culture.

Route Overview:
- The Salkantay Trek typically takes around 4 to 5 days to complete, covering a distance of approximately 70 kilometers (43 miles).
- The trek starts in Mollepata and passes through diverse terrain, including high mountain passes, lush valleys, cloud forests, and eventually descending to Aguas Calientes.
- Trekkers will have the chance to witness breathtaking vistas, including the majestic Salkantay Mountain.

Day 1: Mollepata - Soraypampa:
- Begin the trek in Mollepata and hike to Soraypampa, the first campsite.

- This day includes gradual ascents and offers stunning views of the surrounding mountains.

Day 2: Soraypampa - Salkantay Pass - Chaullay:
- Ascend to the Salkantay Pass at an altitude of about 4,600 meters (15,092 feet), where you'll be rewarded with panoramic views.
- Descend to the cloud forest, passing by the Salkantay River, and camp in Chaullay.

Day 3: Chaullay - La Playa - Lucmabamba:
- Continue through the cloud forest, passing through various ecosystems and local communities.
- Reach the village of La Playa before making your way to Lucmabamba for the night.

Day 4: Lucmabamba - Llactapata - Aguas Calientes:
- Trek to the archaeological site of Llactapata, offering a unique perspective of Machu Picchu from a distance.

- Descend to the Hydroelectric station and continue on foot or take a train to Aguas Calientes.

Day 5: Machu Picchu:
- Begin early to catch the sunrise at Machu Picchu.
- Take a guided tour of the iconic archaeological site and explore its wonders.
- In the afternoon, descend to Aguas Calientes and return to Cusco by train.

Additional Information:
- The Salkantay Trek is considered more challenging than the classic Inca Trail due to the higher altitude and varying terrain.
- The trek does not require a permit, making it a suitable option for those who were unable to secure Inca Trail permits.
- Trekkers can opt to camp or stay in basic lodges along the route, depending on their preferences and the tour package.
- The Salkantay Trek offers a more remote and less crowded experience compared to the classic Inca Trail.

- Weather conditions can vary, so trekkers should be prepared for different temperatures and precipitation.

The Salkantay Trek is a rewarding alternative for those seeking a unique and diverse trekking experience that culminates in the awe-inspiring sight of Machu Picchu.

5.3 Other Trekking Options

In addition to the classic Inca Trail and the Salkantay Trek, there are several other trekking options in the Machu Picchu region that offer unique experiences and stunning landscapes. Here are a few notable alternatives:

1. Lares Trek: The Lares Trek takes you through remote Andean villages and offers interactions with indigenous communities. It's a great way to experience local culture and traditional Andean life. The trek passes by beautiful alpine lakes, hot springs, and offers panoramic views of the surrounding mountains.

2. Choquequirao Trek: This challenging trek leads to the archaeological site of Choquequirao, often referred to as "Machu Picchu's sister site." The site is less visited and provides a sense of exploration and adventure. The trek involves steep ascents and descents, showcasing diverse ecosystems and stunning vistas.

3. Vilcabamba Trek: The Vilcabamba Trek offers a journey through the Vilcabamba Mountain Range, passing by lesser-known archaeological sites and remote villages. The trek provides an opportunity to immerse yourself in the history and culture of the region while enjoying breathtaking views.

4. Ausangate Trek: The Ausangate Trek is known for its high-altitude landscapes and proximity to the Ausangate Mountain, a sacred peak in Andean mythology. Trekkers will pass by vibrant turquoise lakes, traditional communities, and the awe-inspiring Rainbow Mountain.

5. Inca Jungle Trek: The Inca Jungle Trek is a diverse option that combines trekking, mountain biking, and optional activities like zip-lining and rafting. This adventurous route takes you through cloud forests, waterfalls, and ends with a visit to Machu Picchu.

6. Huchuy Qosqo Trek: This shorter trek offers a glimpse into Inca history, leading to the lesser-known archaeological site of Huchuy Qosqo. The trail provides views of the Sacred Valley and the opportunity to learn about the Inca culture.

7. Ampato Trek: The Ampato Trek takes you to the base of Ampato Mountain and offers a visit to the Juanita Mummy, a well-preserved Inca sacrifice found on the mountain. The trek involves hiking through remote landscapes and provides insights into Inca rituals.

CHAPTER SIX
GUIDED TOURS AND INDEPENDENT EXPLORATION

6.1 Pros and Cons of Guided Tours

Guided tours offer a convenient and often enriching way to explore new destinations and cultural attractions like Machu Picchu. However, they may not be suitable for everyone or for every type of travel experience. Here are some pros and cons of guided tours to help you decide whether they are the right choice for your Machu Picchu adventure:

Pros of Guided Tours:

1. Expert Knowledge and Insights: Professional guides provide in-depth knowledge about the history, culture, and significance of the destination, enhancing your understanding and appreciation.

2. Convenience and Logistics: Guided tours handle logistics, such as transportation, accommodations, permits, and entrance

fees, reducing the stress of planning and organizing.

3. Safety and Security: Guides are familiar with the area and its potential challenges, ensuring your safety and well-being during the trip.

4. Local Interactions: Guides can facilitate interactions with locals, providing opportunities to learn about traditional customs and lifestyles.

5. Group Camaraderie: Joining a tour allows you to meet and connect with fellow travelers who share similar interests.

6. Time Efficiency: Guided tours often have optimized itineraries, allowing you to see and experience more within a limited time.

7. Language Barriers: If you're visiting a destination where you're not familiar with the local language, a guide can help bridge the communication gap.

Cons of Guided Tours:

1. Limited Flexibility: Guided tours have fixed schedules and itineraries, limiting your ability to explore at your own pace or make spontaneous changes.

2. Cost: Guided tours may be more expensive than planning and traveling independently, as you're paying for the convenience and services provided.

3. Group Dynamics: The dynamics of a group tour may not suit everyone, and you might have to compromise on certain aspects of your experience.

4. Less Personal Exploration: Guided tours may restrict your opportunities for independent exploration and discovery.

5. Rushed Visits: Due to time constraints and group schedules, guided tours might rush through certain attractions, limiting your time for in-depth exploration.

6. Limited Local Experiences: Depending on the tour, you might have fewer

opportunities to immerse yourself in local life and make personal connections.

7. Tour Quality Variability: The quality of guided tours can vary based on the tour company, guide, and group composition.

Ultimately, the decision to choose a guided tour or to explore independently depends on your travel style, preferences, budget, and comfort level. Some travelers may prefer the convenience and insights offered by guided tours, while others may prioritize the freedom and flexibility of independent travel. It is important to carefully evaluate your options and choose the approach that aligns with your goals for your Machu Picchu experience.

6.2 Tips for Exploring Independently

Exploring Machu Picchu and its surrounding areas independently can be a rewarding and enriching experience. Here are some tips to help you make the most of your independent adventure:

1. Research and Plan Ahead: Research the area, trekking routes, transportation options, and accommodations well in advance to create a detailed itinerary.

2. Secure Permits and Tickets: If you plan to hike the Inca Trail or visit specific sites, ensure you secure the necessary permits and tickets in advance.

3. Acclimatize to Altitude: Spend a few days in Cusco or a nearby town to acclimate to the altitude before embarking on treks or exploring Machu Picchu.

4. Pack Essentials: Pack appropriate clothing for varying weather conditions, sturdy hiking shoes, rain gear, sunscreen, insect repellent, and a refillable water bottle.

5. Navigation: Carry a map, GPS device, or smartphone with navigation apps to help you find your way on trails and in towns.

6. Local Sim Card: Consider getting a local SIM card with data to have access to maps, communication, and emergency assistance.

7. Language Basics: Learn a few basic Spanish phrases to help with communication, as English might not be widely spoken in remote areas.

8. Local Currency: Carry local currency (Peruvian Soles) for transactions, especially in smaller towns and markets.

9. Respect Local Culture: Be respectful of local customs, traditions, and the environment. Follow Leave No Trace principles and respect local communities.

10. Health Precautions: Carry any necessary medications, a basic first aid kit, and stay hydrated to prevent altitude sickness.

11. Flexibility: Embrace flexibility in your plans. Weather, trail conditions, and other factors may require adjustments.

12. Local Transportation: Familiarize yourself with local transportation options, such as buses, minibusses, and trains, to get around efficiently.

13. Interaction with Locals: Engage with locals to learn about their culture, traditions, and recommendations for hidden gems.

14. Emergency Contacts: Have important emergency contacts saved in your phone and share your itinerary with a friend or family member.

15. Photography and Documentation: Capture memories through photography but also take time to immerse yourself in the moment without distractions.

16. Lodging Options: Research accommodations in advance, considering different types (hotels, hostels, lodges) that suit your preferences and budget.

17. Local Cuisine: Sample local dishes and street food to experience authentic Peruvian flavors.

18. Pack Out Waste: Carry out all waste and trash to help preserve the natural beauty of the area.

Exploring independently allows you to create a more personalized and immersive experience. It also requires careful planning and preparation to ensure a safe and enjoyable journey. Embrace the adventure and make the most of your time discovering the wonders of Machu Picchu and its surroundings.

6.3 Hiring Local Guides

Hiring a local guide can greatly enhance your experience when exploring Machu Picchu and its surrounding areas. Local guides provide valuable insights, historical context, and cultural knowledge that can deepen your understanding of the region.

Here are some tips for hiring and working with local guides:

1. Benefits of Hiring a Local Guide:

Expertise: Local guides have in-depth knowledge of the area's history, culture, and attractions, providing you with a more enriching experience.
Cultural Insights: They can share stories, legends, and traditions that may not be found in guidebooks.
Language: Guides can help bridge language barriers and facilitate interactions with locals.
Safety: Local guides are familiar with the terrain, weather conditions, and potential challenges, enhancing your safety.
Supporting the Local Economy: Hiring a local guide directly supports the local community and economy.

2. Finding a Local Guide:

Tour Agencies: Many tour agencies in Cusco and Aguas Calientes offer guided tours to Machu Picchu and other attractions.

Online Platforms: Websites like TripAdvisor, Viator, and GetYourGuide allow you to read reviews and book tours with local guides.

Recommendations: Ask fellow travelers, your accommodations, or locals for recommendations.

3. Qualities to Look for in a Guide:

Knowledgeable: Look for a guide who is knowledgeable about the history, culture, and natural features of the area.

Licensed and Trained: Ensure the guide is licensed and certified by relevant authorities.

Language Skills: Choose a guide who speaks a language you're comfortable with, such as English or Spanish.

Passionate: A passionate guide can make the experience more engaging and memorable.

4. Communication:

Discuss Expectations: Clearly communicate your interests, preferences, and any specific sites you want to visit.

Ask Questions: Don't hesitate to ask questions about the itinerary, timing, transportation, and any concerns you might have.

5. Cost and Tipping:

Negotiate: Negotiate the cost of the tour in advance and ensure you're clear on what's included (transportation, entrance fees, meals, etc.).

Tipping: Tipping is customary in Peru. It's a good practice to tip your guide if you're satisfied with their services.

6. During the Tour:

Engage: Engage with your guide, ask questions, and participate in discussions to make the most of your experience.

Respect Local Customs: Follow your guide's advice regarding local customs, cultural norms, and respectful behavior.

CHAPTER SEVEN
THE MAGNIFICENCE OF MACHU PICCHU

7.1 Arriving at Machu Picchu

Arriving at Machu Picchu is an exciting and awe-inspiring moment, and proper preparation can enhance your experience.

1. Entrance Tickets: Ensure you have your entrance tickets to Machu Picchu. These can be purchased online in advance or in person in Aguas Calientes. Make sure to bring a printed or digital copy of your ticket.

2. Transportation: Most visitors arrive at Machu Picchu from Aguas Calientes, the nearby town. You can reach Aguas Calientes by train from Cusco or Ollantaytambo. From Aguas Calientes, you have the option to take a shuttle bus or hike up to Machu Picchu.

3. Shuttle Bus: Shuttle buses operate between Aguas Calientes and Machu

Picchu. The bus ride takes about 30 minutes and provides scenic views along the way. Buses run frequently in the early morning to accommodate visitors for sunrise.

4. Hiking: If you're up for a hike, you can trek up to Machu Picchu from Aguas Calientes. The hike, known as the "Inca Steps" or "Hiram Bingham Trail," takes around 1.5 to 2 hours. It is recommended to start early to catch the sunrise.

5. Timing: Machu Picchu is open from early morning to late afternoon. The site gets busy, especially during peak tourist seasons, so arriving early in the morning or later in the afternoon can provide a more serene experience.
6. Guided Tours: If you've hired a local guide, they can provide you with insights, historical context, and a guided tour of the site. Guided tours are a great way to fully appreciate the significance of Machu Picchu.

7. Sunrise Experience: Many visitors aim to arrive early to catch the sunrise over Machu Picchu. The site opens its gates around sunrise, and the early morning light creates a magical atmosphere.

8. Essential Items: Bring essentials like a hat, sunscreen, insect repellent, comfortable walking shoes, a refillable water bottle, and your camera to capture the breathtaking views.

9. Visitor Regulations: Follow the guidelines set by the Machu Picchu authorities, such as staying on designated paths, not touching or climbing on the ruins, and respecting the environment.

10. Enjoy the Moment: Take your time to explore and soak in the beauty of Machu Picchu. Find a quiet spot to sit, reflect, and marvel at the impressive architecture and natural surroundings.

11. Departure: Plan your return to Aguas Calientes in time for your departure.

Remember that the last shuttle buses leave Machu Picchu in the late afternoon.

7.2 Layout and Key Structures

Machu Picchu is a remarkable archaeological site with a well-preserved layout and several key structures that hold historical and cultural significance.

Layout:
Machu Picchu is divided into two main areas: the urban sector and the agricultural sector. The urban sector consists of plazas, temples, residential buildings, and ceremonial spaces. The agricultural sector includes terraces, farming areas, and irrigation systems.

Key Structures and Areas:

1. Intihuatana Stone: This granite stone pillar is believed to have been used for astronomical and ritualistic purposes. Its name means "Hitching Post of the Sun."

2. Temple of the Sun (Torreón): This semicircular structure features intricate stonework and is thought to have been a significant religious and astronomical site.

3. Room of the Three Windows: A chamber with three trapezoidal windows overlooking the Urubamba River valley. It's believed to have held ceremonial importance.

4. Main Plaza (Hanan Plaza): A central square where various ceremonies and gatherings may have taken place. It offers stunning views of the surrounding mountains.

5. Royal Tomb (Tumba del Inca): A carved-out rock structure that resembles a tomb. It's unclear whether it was actually a burial site or served another purpose.

6. Sacred Rock (Roca Sagrada): A large rock formation that was likely an important ceremonial site. It is believed to have held religious significance.

7. Residential Areas: Machu Picchu features well-organized residential buildings and living quarters. These structures showcase the impressive Inca stonework and architectural design.

8. Intiwatana Platform: A platform with a carved stone pillar resembling a sundial. It is thought to have been used for astronomical observations and rituals.

9. Guardhouses: These structures are strategically positioned along the site's perimeter. They may have served as lookouts or for defense.

10. Agricultural Terraces: Machu Picchu's well-engineered terraces allowed for farming on the steep slopes. These terraces showcase the Inca's advanced agricultural practices.

11. Inca Trail: The iconic Inca Trail leads to Machu Picchu, passing through diverse landscapes and offering stunning views.

12. Entrance Gate and Watchman's Hut: The entrance gate is where visitors enter Machu Picchu. The Watchman's Hut provides a famous panoramic view of the site.

Machu Picchu's layout and structures reflect the ingenuity and advanced engineering skills of the Inca civilization. Exploring these key areas and structures allows visitors to gain insights into the site's historical, cultural, and architectural significance.

7.3 Sun Gate and Inti Punku

The Sun Gate, known as "Inti Punku" in Quechua, is a significant archaeological site located at Machu Picchu. It holds historical and cultural importance and provides a unique perspective of the ancient citadel. Here's what you need to know about the Sun Gate (Inti Punku):

Location and Purpose: The Sun Gate is situated at the top of a hill overlooking

Machu Picchu. It is strategically positioned along the Inca Trail, which leads to the citadel.

The Inti Punku was likely used as an entrance or checkpoint for those arriving at Machu Picchu via the Inca Trail. It provided a ceremonial and ritualistic entrance to the site.

Features and Characteristics: The Sun Gate consists of a stone structure with a trapezoidal shape, similar to other Inca doorways. It is adorned with precisely cut and fitted stones, showcasing the Inca civilization's advanced stonework techniques. From the Sun Gate, visitors can enjoy breathtaking panoramic views of Machu Picchu, the surrounding mountains, and the Urubamba River valley. The perspective allows for a stunning sight of the entire citadel against its natural backdrop.

Significance: The Sun Gate holds spiritual and astronomical significance. It aligns with the sun's path during the winter solstice, which was an important event for the Inca culture.The name "Inti Punku" translates to "Sun Gate," reflecting its connection to the worship of Inti, the Inca sun god.

Hiking to the Sun Gate: Visitors to Machu Picchu often choose to hike the Inca Trail, which passes through the Sun Gate before descending into the citadel. The hike to the Sun Gate is moderate in difficulty and takes about 1 to 1.5 hours from Machu Picchu's main entrance. It's a popular choice for trekkers looking for an alternative vantage point.

Viewing the Sunrise: While the Sun Gate does not provide the sunrise view of Machu Picchu itself, it offers a unique opportunity to witness the sunrise illuminating the surrounding mountains and the citadel below.

Guided Tours and Interpretation: Many guided tours include a visit to the Sun Gate as part of the Inca Trail trek or a separate hike. Guides often share historical and cultural insights about the Sun Gate, its purpose, and its significance in the Inca civilization.

The Sun Gate (Inti Punku) is not only an architectural marvel but also a place of reverence and connection to the Inca's astronomical and spiritual beliefs. It offers visitors a rewarding and inspiring experience, providing a glimpse into the intricate relationship between Machu Picchu and the natural world.

CHAPTER EIGHT
CULTURAL AND NATURAL HIGHLIGHTS

8.1 Temples and Religious Sites

Machu Picchu is rich with temples and religious sites that provide insights into the spiritual beliefs and practices of the Inca civilization. These structures showcase the Inca's advanced architectural and engineering skills, as well as their deep connection to nature and the cosmos. Here are some notable temples and religious sites within Machu Picchu:

1. Temple of the Sun (Torreón): This semicircular structure is one of the most important religious sites at Machu Picchu. It features precisely cut stones and trapezoidal windows that align with solstices and equinoxes, indicating an astronomical and ceremonial significance. The temple is believed to have been dedicated to the worship of Inti, the sun god.

2. Room of the Three Windows: This chamber contains three trapezoidal windows that offer panoramic views of the surrounding mountains. The room's positioning and architecture suggest it was a ceremonial space where rituals may have taken place, possibly connected to astronomical events.

3. Intiwatana Platform: The Intiwatana is a carved stone pillar resembling a sundial. It is thought to have been used for astronomical observations, particularly related to solstices. The term "Intiwatana" translates to "hitching post of the sun," highlighting its role in connecting the sun to the earth.

4. Main Plaza (Hanan Plaza): The central plaza of Machu Picchu may have been used for various ceremonial and social activities. Its location and layout suggest its importance as a gathering place.

5. Temple of the Condor: This temple is constructed in the shape of a condor, a sacred bird in Inca culture. It features

natural rock formations resembling the condor's wings and body. The temple's layout and symbolism suggest it had spiritual significance.

6. Royal Tomb (Tumba del Inca): Carved into the rock, this structure resembles a tomb, but its exact purpose is debated. It might have held ritualistic or ceremonial significance rather than being an actual burial site.

7. Sacred Rock (Roca Sagrada): A large rock formation that stands near the Main Plaza. It is believed to have held religious importance, possibly as an altar or ceremonial site.

8. Fountains and Water Channels: The complex system of water channels and fountains throughout Machu Picchu may have been used for ritual purification and ceremonial purposes, as water held symbolic significance in Inca culture.

9. Other Temples and Shrines: While not all structures are explicitly labeled as temples,

various other areas within Machu Picchu may have held religious or ceremonial significance. The architectural precision and alignment with astronomical events suggest a deeply spiritual purpose behind their construction.

8.2 Agricultural Terraces

Machu Picchu's agricultural terraces are a remarkable testament to the Inca civilization's advanced engineering and agricultural practices. These terraces served both practical and symbolic purposes, contributing to the sustainability of the site and reflecting the Inca's deep connection to the land.

1. Function: The agricultural terraces were constructed to create flat surfaces on the steep slopes of the Andes mountains. They allowed the Inca to cultivate crops in a challenging and mountainous terrain.

2. Irrigation System: The terraces were designed with a sophisticated irrigation system to distribute water evenly across the

fields. Channels and stone-lined aqueducts brought water from nearby springs and rivers to irrigate the crops.

3. Crop Variety: The Inca cultivated a variety of crops on the terraces, including maize (corn), potatoes, quinoa, beans, and more. The different levels of terraces provided microclimates suitable for various crops.

4. Soil Retention: The terraces also served as a method of preventing soil erosion on the steep slopes. The stone walls held the soil in place and minimized the risk of landslides.

5. Sustainability: The agricultural terraces were an integral part of the Inca's sustainable agricultural practices. They utilized terracing to maximize agricultural output while minimizing the negative impact on the environment.

6. Symbolism: The construction of agricultural terraces was not just practical;

it also held symbolic significance. The stepped terraces represented the Andean concept of "ayni," which emphasizes reciprocity and balance between humans and nature.

7. Alignment with the Cosmos: Some researchers believe that the alignment of certain terraces and agricultural features may have had astronomical or ceremonial purposes, connecting the cultivation of crops with celestial events.

8. Integration with Architecture: The agricultural terraces are seamlessly integrated into the overall layout of Machu Picchu. They provide a stunning backdrop to the architectural structures and enhance the site's aesthetic beauty.

9. Modern Impact: The terraces continue to be a point of interest for visitors, showcasing the Inca's ingenuity and the importance of sustainable agriculture. They also play a role in modern conservation efforts to preserve the site.

8.3 Natural Surroundings and Scenic Views

Machu Picchu's natural surroundings and scenic views are an integral part of its allure and mystique. The site is nestled within the stunning landscapes of the Andes Mountains and offers breathtaking vistas that enhance the overall experience for visitors.

1. Andean Mountains: Machu Picchu is located at an altitude of around 2,430 meters (7,970 feet) above sea level in the Andes Mountains. The surrounding peaks create a dramatic backdrop and contribute to the site's awe-inspiring beauty.

2. Huayna Picchu and Machu Picchu Mountains: These towering peaks frame the citadel, adding to the sense of grandeur. Visitors can hike to the summits of Huayna Picchu or Machu Picchu Mountain for panoramic views of the entire site and the surrounding valleys.

3. Urubamba River Valley: Machu Picchu overlooks the picturesque Urubamba River Valley, offering stunning views of the winding river and lush greenery below.

4. Cloud Forests: The site is enveloped by cloud forests, which contribute to its ethereal atmosphere. The misty and mysterious ambiance adds to the sense of discovery and wonder.

5. Intihuatana Stone Perspective: From the Intihuatana Stone, visitors can enjoy a panoramic view of the entire Machu Picchu complex, including the agricultural terraces, temples, and surrounding landscapes.

6. Sun Gate (Inti Punku) Views: Hiking to the Sun Gate provides an elevated vantage point from which to admire Machu Picchu from a distance, creating a postcard-worthy view of the citadel.

7. Temple of the Sun Overlook: The Temple of the Sun offers a unique view of the Main Plaza and surrounding structures, allowing

you to appreciate the architectural layout and precision of the site.

8. Watchman's Hut Viewpoint: The Watchman's Hut is a famous viewpoint located at the entrance, providing visitors with an iconic view of Machu Picchu with the Huayna Picchu mountain in the background.

9. Sunrise and Sunset: The play of light during sunrise and sunset enhances the magical aura of Machu Picchu. The golden hues against the backdrop of the mountains create unforgettable moments.

10. Serene Beauty: The natural surroundings, including the diverse flora and fauna, contribute to the peaceful and serene ambiance that envelopes the site.

CHAPTER NINE
PHOTOGRAPHY TIPS

9.1 Best Photo Spots

Machu Picchu is a photographer's paradise, offering a multitude of stunning photo spots that capture the site's beauty, history, and natural surroundings.

1. Watchman's Hut Viewpoint: Located near the entrance, this viewpoint offers an iconic panoramic view of Machu Picchu with the Huayna Picchu mountain in the background. It's a popular spot for capturing the entire citadel.

2. Intihuatana Stone: The Intihuatana Stone provides a unique angle to capture the terraces and temples of Machu Picchu in the foreground with the stunning Andean mountains as the backdrop.

3. Sun Gate (Inti Punku): The viewpoint from the Sun Gate offers a picturesque vista of Machu Picchu from a distance. The site is

beautifully framed by the surrounding mountains.

4. Huayna Picchu Summit: If you hike to the summit of Huayna Picchu, you'll be rewarded with breathtaking views of Machu Picchu and the Urubamba River valley from a higher perspective.

5. Machu Picchu Mountain Summit: The Machu Picchu Mountain hike leads to a viewpoint that offers a panoramic view of the entire citadel, showcasing the architectural layout and natural beauty.

6. Temple of the Sun Overlook: Capture the intricate stonework of the Temple of the Sun with the Main Plaza and surrounding structures in the background.

7. Room of the Three Windows: This spot provides a unique angle to capture the ruins and terraces, framed by the trapezoidal windows of the chamber.

8. Agricultural Terraces: Capture the impressive agricultural terraces with their

stone walls and crops, showcasing the Inca's engineering skills against the backdrop of the mountains.

9. Llama Photo Opportunities: Machu Picchu is often visited by llamas and alpacas. Capturing these adorable animals against the ancient ruins creates charming and memorable photos.

10. Sunrise and Sunset: The play of light during sunrise and sunset creates magical photo opportunities. Capture the golden hues as they illuminate the citadel and mountains.

11. Cloud Forest and Misty Atmosphere: Capture the ethereal beauty of Machu Picchu enveloped in mist and surrounded by lush cloud forests.

12. Interaction with Local Culture: Capture candid shots of visitors interacting with local guides, engaging in rituals, or simply taking in the breathtaking surroundings.

9.2 Capturing Sunrise and Sunset

Capturing the sunrise and sunset at Machu Picchu can be a truly magical experience, providing you with breathtaking and atmospheric photos. Here are some tips to help you capture stunning sunrise and sunset shots at this iconic site:

1. Arrive Early: Arrive well before sunrise to secure a good spot and set up your camera. For sunset, plan to be in position about 30 minutes before the sun starts to set.

2. Research Timing: Check the local sunrise and sunset times for the specific date of your visit to ensure you're prepared.

3. Choose a Strategic Location: Plan your location based on where the sun will rise or set in relation to the landscape. The Watchman's Hut or Intihuatana Stone are popular spots for sunrise shots.

4. Bring Essential Gear: Use a sturdy tripod to ensure stability for longer exposures during low light conditions. A wide-angle

lens is also ideal for capturing the expansive views.

5. Shoot in RAW: Capture your photos in RAW format to retain more data for post-processing adjustments.

6. Bracketing for HDR: Consider using bracketing to capture a range of exposures, which can later be merged for high dynamic range (HDR) images.

7. Manual Mode: Use manual mode to have full control over your camera settings, including shutter speed, aperture, and ISO.

8. Set a Low ISO: Use a low ISO setting to minimize noise and ensure clean images.

9. Use a Small Aperture: A smaller aperture (higher f-number) will help ensure a larger depth of field, keeping both foreground and background in focus.

10. Graduated ND Filters: If the dynamic range is too high, use graduated neutral density (ND) filters to balance the exposure

between the bright sky and darker foreground.

11. Experiment with Compositions: Try different compositions, framing the ancient ruins against the colorful sky. Include interesting foreground elements to add depth.

12. Long Exposures (Optional): For creative effects, you can experiment with long exposures to capture the movement of clouds or water (if applicable).

13. Post-Processing: In post-processing, fine-tune the exposure, color balance, and contrast to bring out the best in your sunrise or sunset shots.

14. Be Patient and Enjoy the Moment: While capturing the perfect shot is important, remember to take moments to simply appreciate the stunning beauty of the sunrise or sunset over Machu Picchu.

9.3 Recommend Gear

When visiting Machu Picchu, having the right gear can greatly enhance your experience and help you capture memorable moments. Here's a recommended list of gear to consider bringing with you:

1. Camera: A digital camera with manual settings (DSLR or mirrorless) will give you more control over your photos, but a high-quality smartphone can also produce great results.

2. Lenses: Wide-angle lenses (10-24mm) are ideal for capturing the expansive views and grandeur of Machu Picchu. A telephoto lens (70-200mm) can be useful for capturing details and compressing the perspective.

3. Tripod: A sturdy tripod is essential for capturing stable shots, especially during low light conditions such as sunrise and sunset.

4. Extra Batteries and Memory Cards: Ensure you have enough power and storage space for your camera. Machu Picchu's mesmerizing views might lead to taking more photos than anticipated.

5. Lens Cleaning Kit: The misty atmosphere of Machu Picchu can sometimes lead to condensation on your lens. A cleaning kit will help you maintain clear shots.

6. Filters: Consider bringing polarizing filters to enhance colors and reduce reflections, and graduated neutral density (ND) filters to balance exposure between the sky and landscape.

7. Camera Bag or Backpack: Choose a comfortable and weather-resistant bag to carry your camera gear and other essentials.

8. Rain Protection: Rain is common in the region, especially during certain seasons. Bring a rain cover for your camera and backpack to protect your gear.

9. Smartphone: A smartphone with a good camera can be a convenient backup for quick shots and sharing moments in real-time.

10. Portable Charger: Keep your devices charged throughout the day with a portable charger or power bank.

11. Comfortable Shoes and Clothing: Wear comfortable walking shoes with good grip for exploring the site. Dress in layers to accommodate changing weather conditions.

12. Hat and Sunglasses: Protect yourself from the sun's rays while exploring the site.

13. Sunscreen and Insect Repellent: Stay protected from the sun and insects, especially if you plan to spend extended periods outdoors.

14. Water Bottle: Stay hydrated by carrying a refillable water bottle. There are water refill stations available at Machu Picchu.

15. Snacks: Pack light, energizing snacks to keep you fueled during your exploration.

16. Personal Identification and Tickets: Carry a valid form of identification and your entrance tickets to Machu Picchu.

17. Notebook and Pen: Jot down notes, observations, or thoughts about your experience.

CHAPTER TEN
RESPECTING THE SITE

10.1 Sustainable Tourism Practices

Engaging in sustainable tourism practices at Machu Picchu is essential to help preserve the site's natural and cultural heritage for future generations.

1. Respect Local Culture: Learn about and respect the local customs, traditions, and etiquette of the region. Engage with local communities in a culturally sensitive manner.

2. Choose Responsible Tour Operators: Opt for tour operators and guides that prioritize sustainability, support local communities, and follow ethical practices.

3. Pack Out What You Bring In: Carry reusable water bottles and containers, and avoid single-use plastics. Properly dispose of your waste in designated bins or take it with you.

4. Minimize Plastic Usage: Refrain from purchasing single-use plastic items such as water bottles and straws. Use eco-friendly alternatives.

5. Reduce Energy Consumption: Conserve energy by turning off lights, air conditioning, and other electrical devices when not in use.

6. Support Local Economy: Purchase locally made crafts, products, and souvenirs to support the livelihoods of local artisans and communities.

7. Use Water Wisely: Be mindful of water usage and take shorter showers. Follow any water conservation guidelines set by accommodations.

8. Choose Eco-Friendly Accommodations: Stay in accommodations that have sustainability initiatives, such as energy-efficient practices and waste reduction.

9. Opt for Responsible Transportation: Choose eco-friendly transportation options, such as trains or buses, over private vehicles. If you must travel by car, consider carpooling.

10. Respect Wildlife and Nature: Do not disturb or feed wildlife, and refrain from picking plants or damaging the environment. Stay on designated trails to minimize your impact.

11. Cultural Sensitivity: Dress modestly when visiting cultural or religious sites, and ask for permission before taking photos of people.

12. Opt for Group Tours: Group tours generally have a lower environmental impact than individual tours, as they use shared resources more efficiently.

13. Stay Informed: Educate yourself about the site's rules and regulations. Follow guidelines provided by authorities to protect the site and its surroundings.

14. Leave No Trace: Follow the principles of "Leave No Trace" by leaving the environment as you found it. Avoid leaving behind any trash or impact.

15. Participate in Conservation Efforts: Consider volunteering or participating in conservation initiatives that contribute to the protection and preservation of Machu Picchu.

10.2 Leave No Trace Principles

The "Leave No Trace" principles provide a set of guidelines to minimize your impact on the environment while enjoying outdoor and natural spaces. When visiting places like Machu Picchu, it's important to follow these principles to help preserve the site's natural and cultural heritage. Here are the seven "Leave No Trace" principles:

1. Plan Ahead and Prepare: Research and understand the regulations, weather, and terrain of the area you're visiting. Plan your

trip to minimize the need for excessive resources and avoid overcrowding.

2. Travel and Camp on Durable Surfaces: Stick to designated trails and established campsites. Avoid trampling on vegetation and fragile ecosystems. When visiting archaeological sites like Machu Picchu, stay on designated paths to protect the ruins.

3. Dispose of Waste Properly: Pack out all trash, leftover food, and litter. Use designated restroom facilities when available. At Machu Picchu, follow waste disposal guidelines and use provided trash receptacles.

4. Leave What You Find: Avoid picking plants, disturbing wildlife, or altering the environment in any way. Preserve the site's natural and cultural features for others to enjoy.

5. Minimize Campfire Impact: Use a camp stove for cooking instead of making campfires, especially in sensitive areas.

Fires can cause lasting damage to ecosystems and archaeological sites.

6. Respect Wildlife: Observe animals from a distance and avoid feeding them. Human food can be harmful to wildlife and alter their natural behaviors.

7. Be Considerate of Other Visitors: Keep noise levels down, yield the trail to others, and maintain a respectful distance from other visitors. At popular sites like Machu Picchu, practice patience and courteous behavior.

10.3 Cultural Sensitivity

Cultural sensitivity is the awareness, understanding, and respectful consideration of the beliefs, customs, traditions, and values of different cultures. When visiting a place as culturally significant as Machu Picchu, it's crucial to approach the experience with cultural sensitivity to ensure that you respect the local heritage, customs, and the environment.

1. Learn About the Local Culture: Educate yourself about the history, traditions, and customs of the Inca civilization and the local communities in the region.

2. Dress Modestly: When visiting sacred sites or interacting with local communities, dress modestly and respectfully. Avoid clothing that may be considered inappropriate or offensive.

3. Ask for Permission: Before taking photos of people, especially locals, always ask for permission. Respect their wishes if they decline.

4. Engage with Respect: Interact with locals and guides respectfully, using appropriate language and demeanor. Show genuine interest and appreciation for their culture.

5. Follow Site Guidelines: Follow the rules and regulations set by the authorities at Machu Picchu. These guidelines are in

place to protect the site and its cultural heritage.

6. Leave No Trace: Practice "Leave No Trace" principles to ensure you leave the site as you found it, respecting the environment and the cultural significance of the area.

7. Participate Thoughtfully: If you choose to participate in cultural activities or rituals, do so with sincerity and an open mind. Avoid treating such experiences as mere photo opportunities.

8. Respect Personal Space: Be mindful of personal space and boundaries, both with other visitors and with locals. Respect social norms and customs.

9. Support Local Economy: Purchase locally made crafts and products to support the local economy and communities.

10. Avoid Stereotyping: Avoid making assumptions or generalizations about the

local culture or people based on stereotypes.

11. Listen and Learn: Engage in meaningful conversations with locals and guides to gain insights into their culture, history, and way of life.

12. Be Humble and Curious: Approach your visit with humility and a genuine desire to learn about and understand the cultural significance of Machu Picchu.

13. Mindful Photography: When taking photos, be mindful of cultural sensitivities. Avoid photographing sacred rituals or private moments without permission.

14. Support Sustainable Tourism: Choose tour operators and practices that prioritize cultural preservation, environmental sustainability, and benefit local communities.

CHAPTER ELEVEN
ADDITIONAL ATTRACTIONS NEARBY

11.1 Huayna Picchu Hike

Huayna Picchu, often spelled as Wayna Picchu, is the iconic mountain that towers above Machu Picchu, offering spectacular panoramic views of the ancient citadel and its surrounding landscapes. Hiking Huayna Picchu is a popular and rewarding experience for visitors seeking a different perspective of Machu Picchu.

1. Permits and Reservations: Access to Huayna Picchu is limited, and a separate entrance ticket is required. It's recommended to secure your permit well in advance, as availability is limited.

2. Hiking Difficulty: The hike is considered moderately strenuous and involves steep sections, narrow paths, and some exposed areas. It's not recommended for those with a fear of heights or limited mobility.

3. Trail Duration: The hike typically takes about 1.5 to 2.5 hours to reach the summit, depending on your pace and fitness level.

4. Trailhead and Start Time: The trailhead for the Huayna Picchu hike is near the entrance to Machu Picchu. There are two entry time slots for the hike: one at 7:00 AM and another at 10:00 AM. Choose the time slot that suits your preference.

5. Scenic Views: The highlight of the hike is reaching the summit, where you'll be rewarded with breathtaking views of Machu Picchu from above. You'll also have panoramic vistas of the surrounding mountains and valleys.

6. Temple of the Moon: Along the trail, you'll come across the Temple of the Moon, an ancient Inca shrine built into a cave. This adds to the historical and archaeological significance of the hike.

7. Limited Capacity: Due to its popularity and the need to preserve the environment, the number of hikers allowed on Huayna

Picchu each day is restricted. This enhances the experience by reducing crowding.

8. Safety Precautions: As with any hike, wear appropriate footwear and clothing, bring sufficient water and snacks, and be prepared for changing weather conditions.

9. Guided Tours: Some visitors choose to join guided tours that include the Huayna Picchu hike as part of the itinerary. Guides can provide insights into the history and significance of the mountain.

10. Age and Fitness Requirements: While the hike is manageable for many, it may not be suitable for young children or those with certain health conditions. It's important to assess your own fitness level and consult with medical professionals if needed.

11.2 Machu Picchu Mountain Hike

The Machu Picchu Mountain hike is another popular trekking option for visitors to Machu Picchu, offering stunning panoramic views of the citadel and its surrounding landscapes.

1. Permits and Reservations: Similar to Huayna Picchu, a separate entrance ticket is required for the Machu Picchu Mountain hike, and permits are limited. It's advisable to secure your permit well in advance.

2. Hiking Difficulty: The hike to Machu Picchu Mountain is considered challenging and involves steep ascents and descents. It's recommended for those who are physically fit and have some hiking experience.

3. Trail Duration: The hike typically takes about 3 to 4 hours to reach the summit, depending on your pace and rest stops.

4. Trailhead and Start Time: The trailhead for the Machu Picchu Mountain hike is located near the entrance to Machu Picchu. There are two entry time slots for the hike: one at 7:00 AM and another at 9:00 AM.

5. Scenic Views: The primary attraction of the Machu Picchu Mountain hike is the breathtaking panoramic view from the summit. You will have a bird's-eye perspective of Machu Picchu, the Urubamba River valley, and the surrounding mountains.

6. Less Crowded: Compared to Huayna Picchu, Machu Picchu Mountain sees fewer hikers, allowing for a quieter and more serene experience.

7. Natural Beauty: The hike takes you through lush cloud forests, providing opportunities to observe local flora and fauna.

8. Fitness Level: The hike is physically demanding, with steep inclines and uneven terrain. Be prepared for a challenging ascent.

9. Safety Precautions: As with any hike, wear appropriate footwear and clothing, bring sufficient water and snacks, and be prepared for changing weather conditions.

10. Guided Tours: Many guided tours include the Machu Picchu Mountain hike as part of their itinerary. Guides can provide valuable insights into the natural and cultural aspects of the area.

11. Age and Fitness Requirements: Due to the challenging nature of the hike, it's important to assess your own fitness level and consult with medical professionals if needed.

12. Consider Combination with Machu Picchu Visit: Some visitors choose to combine the Machu Picchu Mountain hike with a visit to the main citadel. This provides a comprehensive exploration of the site.

11.3 Hot Springs at Aguas Calientes

Aguas Calientes, the gateway town to Machu Picchu, is known for its natural hot springs that offer a relaxing and rejuvenating experience for visitors.

1. Location: The hot springs are located a short distance from the center of Aguas Calientes, making them easily accessible for visitors.

2. Thermal Waters: The hot springs feature thermal waters rich in minerals, which are believed to have therapeutic properties. The temperature of the pools can vary, offering options for both warm and hot baths.

3. Relaxation and Healing: Many people visit the hot springs to unwind and relax after exploring Machu Picchu or engaging in trekking activities. The warm waters are thought to provide relaxation and relief to tired muscles.

4. Spectacular Setting: The hot springs are surrounded by lush greenery and the natural beauty of the Andean landscape, creating a tranquil and picturesque environment.

5. Bathing Experience: The hot springs typically have a series of pools with varying temperatures. Visitors can soak in the mineral-rich waters while enjoying the views.

6. Local Culture: The hot springs are also a place where you can interact with locals and other travelers, making it a social and cultural experience.

7. Amenities: The hot springs area may include changing rooms, showers, and other facilities to enhance your bathing experience.

8. Timing and Crowds: The hot springs can get busy, especially during peak tourist seasons. Consider visiting during non-peak hours to avoid crowds.

9. Bring Essentials: Bring a swimsuit, towel, and any personal toiletries you may need.

10. Respect the Environment: While enjoying the hot springs, be mindful of your impact on the environment. Follow any

guidelines provided by the hot springs facility.

CHAPTER TWELVE
PRACTICAL INFORMATION

12.1 Safety and Health Considerations

When visiting Machu Picchu and its surrounding areas, ensuring your safety and health is of utmost importance. Here are some key safety and health considerations to keep in mind:

1. Altitude Sickness: Machu Picchu is situated at a high altitude, which can lead to altitude sickness (also known as acute mountain sickness). Give yourself time to acclimatize by spending a day or two in Cusco or other lower-altitude areas before heading to Machu Picchu.

2. Hydration and Nutrition: Stay hydrated by drinking plenty of water and consuming electrolyte-rich beverages. Maintain a balanced diet to support your energy levels during hikes and exploration.

3. Sun Protection: The high altitude and strong sun can lead to sunburn and dehydration. Wear sunscreen, sunglasses, and a wide-brimmed hat. Use lip balm with SPF protection.

4. Proper Clothing and Footwear: Wear appropriate clothing for varying weather conditions, including rain and sun. Comfortable and sturdy footwear with good grip is essential for exploring the site and hiking.

5. Insect Protection: In certain areas, insects can be a nuisance. Use insect repellent to protect against bites.

6. Stay on Designated Paths: Follow marked trails and designated paths to avoid getting lost and minimize your impact on the environment.

7. Personal Safety: Be cautious when walking on uneven terrain, especially around archaeological sites. Pay attention to your surroundings and exercise caution when taking photos near ledges or edges.

8. Emergency Contacts: Have emergency contact numbers handy, including local authorities, medical facilities, and your country's embassy or consulate.

9. First Aid Kit: Carry a basic first aid kit with essentials such as bandages, antiseptic wipes, pain relievers, and any personal medications.

10. Travel Insurance: Purchase travel insurance that covers medical emergencies, trip cancellations, and other unforeseen events.

11. Respect Local Customs: Be respectful of local customs, traditions, and etiquette. Ask for permission before taking photos of people, especially locals.

12. Wildlife Safety: If you encounter wildlife, maintain a safe distance and avoid feeding or approaching animals.

13. Secure Your Belongings: Keep your valuables secure and be cautious of pickpocketing, especially in crowded areas.

14. Group Tours: Consider joining guided tours, especially for hikes and treks, as they often provide safety measures, local insights, and assistance in case of emergencies.

12.2 Language and Communication

Language and communication are essential aspects of any travel experience, including when visiting Machu Picchu and its surrounding areas.

1. Official Languages: The official languages of Peru are Spanish and Quechua, the latter being the language of the Inca civilization. While Spanish is widely spoken, especially in urban areas, some locals, particularly in rural communities, may primarily speak Quechua.

2. English Proficiency: In tourist areas like Machu Picchu and Aguas Calientes, you'll find that many locals, guides, and service providers have a basic to moderate level of English proficiency. However, it's helpful to learn a few basic phrases in Spanish or Quechua to enhance your interactions.

3. Basic Phrases: Learning a few key phrases in the local language can go a long way in making connections and showing respect to the local culture. Phrases such as greetings, thank you, and asking for directions can be especially useful.

4. Language Apps and Guides: Language apps and pocket guides can be valuable resources for on-the-go translation and communication assistance.

5. Local Guides: Hiring a local guide who is fluent in English or your native language can enhance your understanding of the cultural and historical significance of Machu Picchu.

6. Communication Challenges: In remote areas or less touristy locations, you may encounter limited English-speaking individuals. Be patient and use non-verbal communication, gestures, and visual aids to convey your needs.

7. Respectful Communication: Approach conversations with respect and an open-minded attitude. Embrace the opportunity to learn about the local culture through meaningful interactions.

8. Written Information: Many signs, brochures, and information boards at popular tourist sites are available in multiple languages, including English.

9. Language Barriers and Connection: Do not let language barriers discourage you from exploring. Often, the warmth and friendliness of the locals can transcend verbal communication.

10. Cultural Sensitivity: Be aware of cultural nuances in communication, such as

greetings and body language, to avoid misunderstandings.

11. Offline Translation Apps: Consider using offline translation apps that allow you to translate phrases even when you don't have internet access.

12. Learn the Basics: While fluency isn't necessary, learning a bit about the local language and culture can enrich your experience and show your respect for the destination.

13. Interact with Locals: Engage with locals in a friendly and open manner, and you'll likely find that they appreciate your effort to communicate.

12.3 Currency and Banking

When traveling to Machu Picchu and Peru, understanding the local currency and banking options is important for a smooth and convenient trip.

Currency: The official currency of Peru is the Peruvian Sol (S/), often symbolized as "S/." Coins are available in various denominations, including 5, 10, 20, and 50 centimos, as well as 1, 2, and 5 soles.Banknotes are available in denominations of 10, 20, 50, 100, and 200 soles.

Currency Exchange: It is recommended to exchange currency upon arrival at the airport or in major cities like Lima or Cusco. Exchange rates may vary, so compare rates before exchanging money. Banks, exchange bureaus (casas de cambio), and authorized currency exchange offices are common throughout tourist areas.

ATMs: ATMs (cajeros automáticos) are widely available in cities and towns, including Aguas Calientes (the gateway to Machu Picchu). Use ATMs affiliated with well-known banks to ensure security and reliable exchange rates. Keep in mind that some remote areas may have limited ATM access, so it is advisable to withdraw cash in larger towns before traveling to such places.

Credit Cards: Credit cards (Visa, MasterCard, and to a lesser extent, American Express) are widely accepted in larger cities, upscale restaurants, hotels, and tour agencies. In more remote areas, cash may be the preferred form of payment, so it's a good idea to have both cash and cards on hand.

Currency Tips: Notify your bank about your travel plans to avoid any issues with card transactions. Keep small bills for small purchases, as some places may not have change for larger denominations. Carry some US dollars as a backup, as they are sometimes accepted in tourist areas.

Tipping: Tipping is customary in Peru. In restaurants, a service charge (propina) may be included in the bill, but it's common to leave an additional tip of 5-10% for good service. Tipping for tour guides, drivers, and hotel staff is also appreciated.

Currency Conversion: As currency exchange rates can fluctuate, it's a good idea to use a reliable currency conversion app or website to check current rates before making transactions.

Safety: When using ATMs or exchanging money, be cautious of your surroundings and ensure your personal information is protected.

12.4 Useful Phrases

Learning a few basic phrases in the local language can greatly enhance your travel experience and interactions with locals in Machu Picchu and Peru. Here are some useful phrases in Spanish that you might find helpful:

Greetings and Polite Expressions:
- Hello: Hola
- Good morning: Buenos días
- Good afternoon/evening: Buenas tardes
- Good night: Buenas noches
- Please: Por favor

- Thank you: Gracias
- You're welcome: De nada
- Excuse me/pardon me: Perdón/disculpe

Basic Communication:
- Yes: Sí
- No: No
- Maybe: Tal vez
- I don't understand: No entiendo
- Can you help me?: ¿Puede ayudarme?
- How much does this cost?: ¿Cuánto cuesta esto?
- Where is...?: ¿Dónde está...?
- What is your name?: ¿Cuál es su nombre?
- My name is...: Mi nombre es...
- I'm from...: Soy de...

Numbers:
- One: Uno
- Two: Dos
- Three: Tres
- Four: Cuatro
- Five: Cinco
- Ten: Diez
- Twenty: Veinte
- Hundred: Cien
- Thousand: Mil

Directions:
- Left: Izquierda
- Right: Derecha
- Straight ahead: Todo recto
- Where is the bathroom?: ¿Dónde está el baño?
- Can you show me on a map?: ¿Puede mostrarme en un mapa?

Food and Dining:
- Menu: Carta/menú
- Water: Agua
- Breakfast: Desayuno
- Lunch: Almuerzo
- Dinner: Cena
- I'm vegetarian/vegan: Soy vegetariano/vegano
- Check, please: La cuenta, por favor

Emergency and Health:
- Help!: ¡Ayuda!
- Doctor: Médico
- Pharmacy: Farmacia
- I need a hospital: Necesito un hospital
- I'm not feeling well: No me siento bien

Remember, making an effort to communicate in the local language, even if it's just a few phrases, can show respect for the culture and enhance your interactions with locals. Most Peruvians appreciate when visitors try to communicate in Spanish, and your efforts are likely to be met with warmth and friendliness.

CHAPTER THIRTEEN
RESOURCES AND CONTACTS

13.1 Travel agencies and tour operators

When planning a trip to Machu Picchu, engaging with reputable travel agencies and tour operators can help ensure a well-organized and enjoyable experience. These professionals can assist with transportation, accommodations, guided tours, permits, and more. Here are some notable travel agencies and tour operators that offer services for Machu Picchu and its surrounding areas:

1. Peru Rail: The official train operator to Machu Picchu, offering various train services from Cusco and Ollantaytambo to Aguas Calientes.

2. Inca Rail: Another train operator offering services to Machu Picchu, with options for different budgets and travel preferences.

3. Machu Picchu Tours: A local agency specializing in Machu Picchu tours and treks, providing a range of guided experiences.

4. Intrepid Travel: Offers a variety of small group tours to Machu Picchu, combining cultural experiences and outdoor adventures.

5. G Adventures: Known for responsible and sustainable travel, G Adventures offers guided tours that include Machu Picchu and other highlights.

6. Llama Path: A well-regarded agency specializing in Inca Trail treks, including options for various trekking routes.

7. Peru Treks and Adventure: Offers guided tours and treks to Machu Picchu, including the Inca Trail and alternative routes.

8. Enigma Peru: Offers luxury and premium tours to Machu Picchu, focusing on high-quality service and unique experiences.

9. Kuoda Travel: A boutique travel agency offering personalized itineraries and private tours to Machu Picchu and other Peruvian destinations.

10. Andean Adventures: Specializes in sustainable and eco-friendly tours to Machu Picchu, emphasizing cultural exchange and community engagement.

11. Explorandes: Offers a range of guided tours and treks to Machu Picchu, with a focus on cultural immersion and outdoor exploration.

When choosing a travel agency or tour operator, it is important to consider factors such as their reputation, reviews from past travelers, the quality of their services, their commitment to sustainable and responsible tourism practices, and the specific itineraries they offer. Whichever agency you choose, make sure they are licensed and authorized to operate in the region, and communicate your preferences and needs clearly to ensure a tailored and memorable experience at Machu Picchu.

13.2 Official Websites and Resources

When planning a trip to Machu Picchu, it's important to rely on official and reliable resources to ensure accurate and up-to-date information.

1. Ministry of Culture of Peru - Machu Picchu: The official government website provides information about Machu Picchu, its history, regulations, and visitor guidelines.

Website: https://www.machupicchu.gob.pe/

2. Peru Tourism Board (PromPeru): The official tourism board of Peru offers comprehensive information about travel destinations, activities, and practical travel tips.

Website: https://www.peru.travel/

3. National Institute of Culture (INC): Provides information about cultural heritage, archaeological sites, and preservation efforts in Peru.
Website: https://inc.pe/

4. Peru Rail: The official website for train services to Machu Picchu, including routes, schedules, and ticket booking.
Website: https://www.perurail.com/

5. Inca Rail: Another official train operator to Machu Picchu, offering various travel options and services.
Website: https://incarail.com/

6. Official Inca Trail Regulations: Learn about the regulations and guidelines for hiking the Inca Trail to Machu Picchu, including permit information.
Website: http://www.incatrail.gob.pe/

7. Cusco Tourist Information: The official tourism website for Cusco provides details about attractions, accommodations, and activities in the region.

Website: https://www.cuscotourismoffice.com/

8. Aguas Calientes Municipal Website: Offers information about Aguas Calientes, including accommodations, transportation, and services.
Website: http://www.muniaguas.com/

9. U.S. Embassy & Consulate in Peru: Provides travel advisories, safety information, and resources for U.S. citizens traveling to Peru.
Website: https://pe.usembassy.gov/

10. Lonely Planet - Machu Picchu: A reliable travel resource with information, tips, and travel guides for visiting Machu Picchu.
Website: https://www.lonelyplanet.com/peru/machu-picchu

It is expedient to cross-reference information from multiple official sources and reputable travel guides to ensure accuracy and reliability. These resources will help you plan a safe and memorable trip to Machu Picchu while staying informed about regulations, cultural practices, and logistics.

13.3 Emergency Contacts

When traveling to Machu Picchu and Peru, it is important to have access to emergency contacts in case you need assistance. Here are some key emergency contacts to keep handy during your trip:

Emergency Services:
- Police: 105
- Medical Emergency: 116
- Fire Department: 116

Tourist Police: The Tourist Police (Policía de Turismo) specialize in assisting tourists and can help with a range of issues including theft, lost items, and emergencies.
Tourist Police Emergency: 0800-22221

Medical Assistance: SAMU (Medical Emergency Service): 106
Hospitals and Medical Facilities: Research and note down the nearest hospitals and medical facilities in the areas you're visiting.

Embassies and Consulates: Contact your country's embassy or consulate in case of emergencies or if you require assistance with lost documents, legal matters, or other issues.

U.S. Embassy & Consulate in Peru:
Website: https://pe.usembassy.gov/
Emergency Contact: +51-1-618-2000 (For U.S. citizens)

Canadian Embassy & Consulates in Peru:
Website:
https://www.canadainternational.gc.ca/per u/index.aspx?lang=eng
Emergency Contact: +51-1-319-3200 (For Canadians)

UK Embassy & Consulate in Peru:

Website:
https://www.gov.uk/world/organisations/
british-embassy-lima
Emergency Contact: +51-1-617-3000 (For
British nationals)

Australian Embassy & Consulate in Peru:
Website: https://peru.embassy.gov.au/
Emergency Contact: +51-1-630-0500 (For
Australians)

New Zealand Honorary Consulate in Peru:
Contact: antonia.garcia@mfat.govt.nz (For
New Zealanders)

Local Tour Operator or Hotel:
Keep the contact information of your local
tour operator, guide, or hotel reception
handy in case you need assistance or
information during your stay.

Insurance Provider:
If you have travel insurance, keep your
insurance provider's contact information
easily accessible.

It is good to store these emergency contacts in your phone and keep a physical copy in your travel documents. While emergencies are rare, being prepared with the right contacts can provide peace of mind and ensure that you can quickly access help if needed.

Appendix
Recommended Reading and Films

Engaging with literature and films related to Machu Picchu can deepen your understanding of its history, culture, and significance. Below are some recommended reading and films that can enhance your experience:

Books:

1. "Turn Right at Machu Picchu" by Mark Adams:
A modern travelogue that follows the author's journey along the Inca Trail and his exploration of the history and mysteries surrounding Machu Picchu.

2. "The Last Days of the Incas" by Kim MacQuarrie:
This historical account provides insights into the fall of the Inca Empire and the events leading up to the Spanish conquest, including the story of Machu Picchu.

3. "Machu Picchu: A Civil Engineering Marvel" by Ken Wright:

A detailed exploration of the engineering and architectural aspects of Machu Picchu, highlighting its sophisticated construction techniques.

4. "The Conquest of the Incas"by John Hemming:

An authoritative history of the Spanish conquest of the Inca Empire, shedding light on the broader context of Machu Picchu's creation.

5. "The White Rock: An Exploration of the Inca Heartland" by Hugh Thomson:

This travel memoir delves into the author's journey through the Andes, visiting Machu Picchu and other Inca sites, while reflecting on history and culture.

Films and Documentaries:

1. "The Secret of the Incas" (1954):

Often cited as an inspiration for the Indiana Jones series, this adventure film starring Charlton Heston features Machu Picchu and explores Inca archaeology.

2. "The Great Inca Rebellion" (2010):
A documentary that examines the story of the Inca rebellion against Spanish rule, shedding light on the events leading up to the fall of the empire and the impact on Machu Picchu.

3. "Machu Picchu Decoded" (2012):
A National Geographic documentary that delves into the mysteries and history of Machu Picchu, exploring its construction, purpose, and cultural significance.

4. "The Inca: Masters of the Clouds" (2015):
A documentary series that provides a comprehensive look at the Inca civilization, including their achievements, beliefs, and the construction of Machu Picchu.

5. "Machu Picchu: The Deciphering of the Stones" (2016):
An educational documentary that explores the architectural and engineering

marvels of Machu Picchu, revealing the techniques used in its construction.

These books and films offer diverse perspectives on Machu Picchu and the Inca civilization, allowing you to delve deeper into the history, culture, and significance of this iconic site. They can enrich your travel experience by providing context and insights into the world you'll be exploring.

Printed in Great Britain
by Amazon

44243102R00089